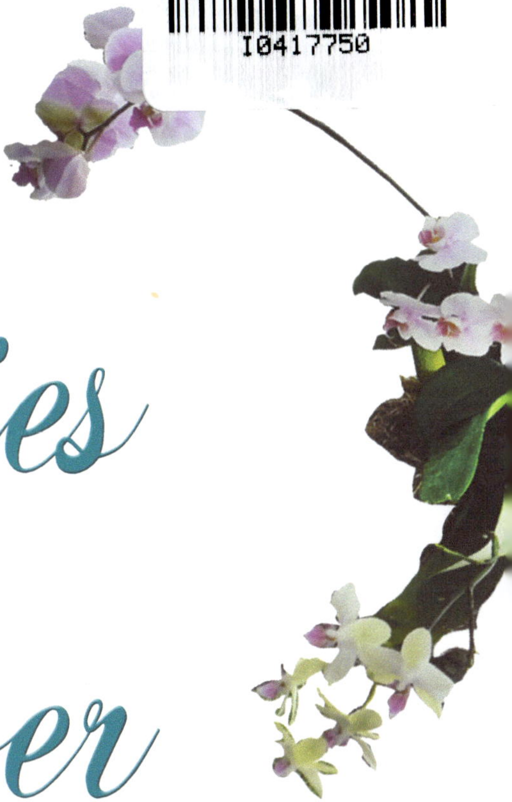

Memories of a Caregiver

BY

DAVID MITCHELL

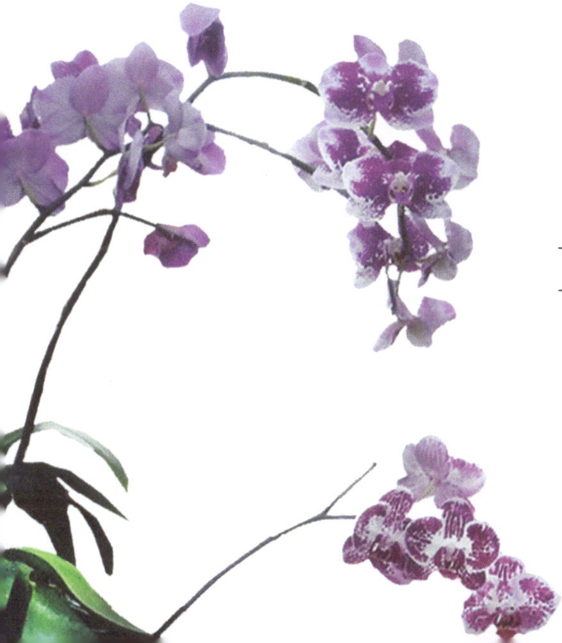

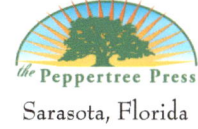

the Peppertree Press

Sarasota, Florida

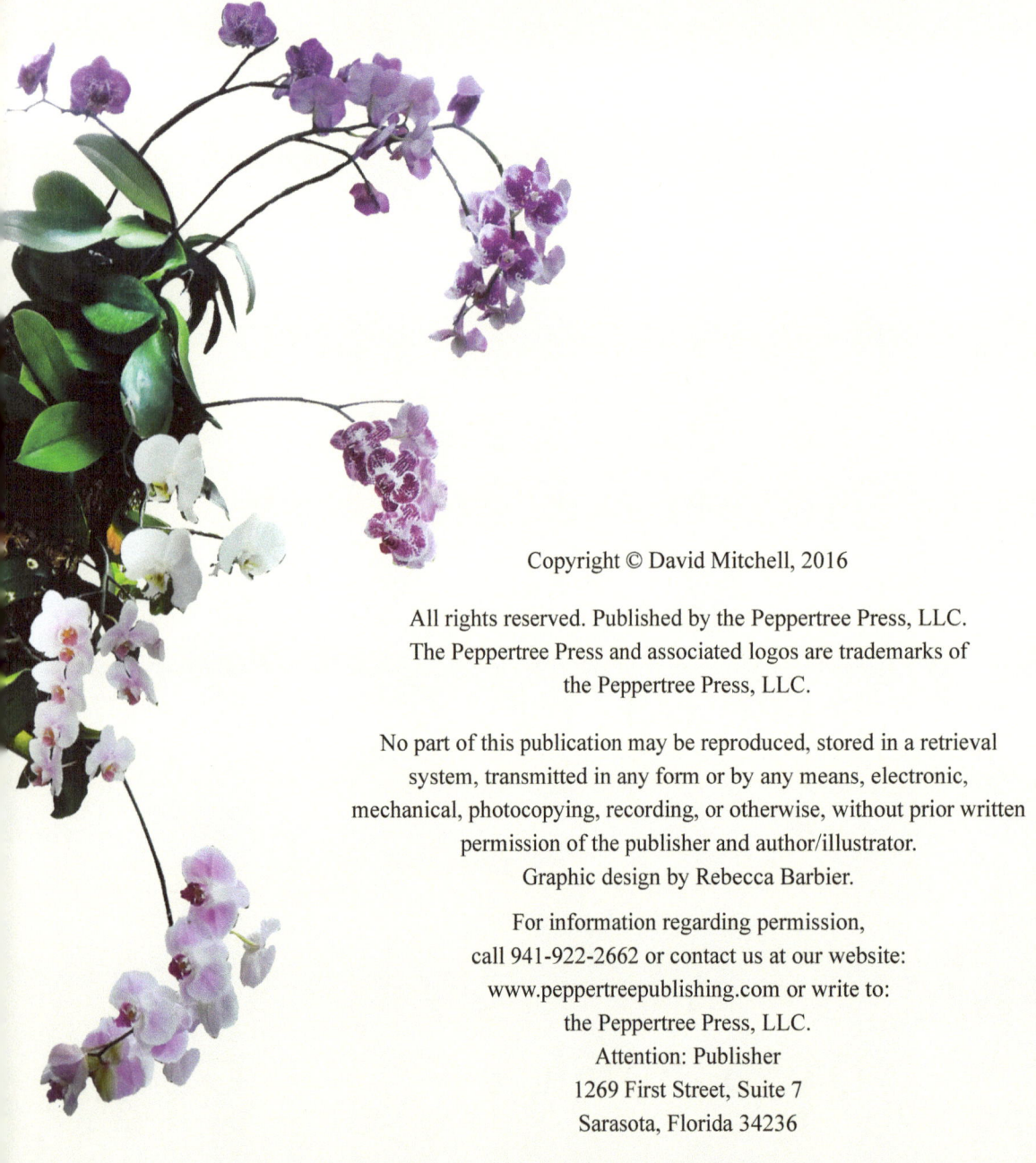

For information regarding permission,
call 941-922-2662 or contact us at our website:
www.peppertreepublishing.com or write to:
the Peppertree Press, LLC.
Attention: Publisher
1269 First Street, Suite 7
Sarasota, Florida 34236

ISBN: 978-1-61493-491-2

Library of Congress Number: 2016919296

Printed January 2017

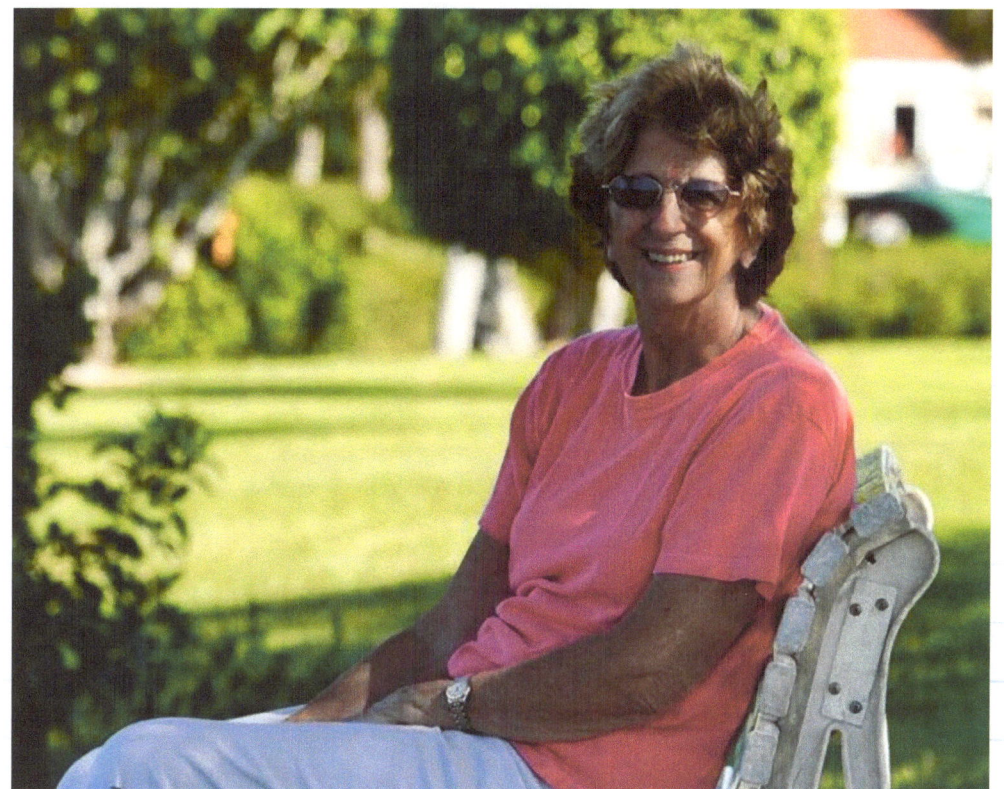

Kathy at her best, 2006

My wife, Kathy, died on October 10th, 2015 after many years of sinking into Alzheimer's disease. The disease began with minor forgetfulness, vaguely noticeable around 2007, and my earliest attempt to get some kind of action going led to a near-disastrous family battle.

When I told her, as we drove to a doctor's appointment, that I was planning to tell our doctor about my concern for Kathy's memory, she told me, in no uncertain terms that I was not to do so. I insisted that it was my duty and responsibility to see if there was anything that could be done about it. When I made my report, the doctor put us in touch with more than one neurologist.

During a visit of one of Kathy's sisters, Kathy reported my 'cruelty' in reporting her memory problems to the doctor, whereupon her sister attacked me forcefully. I defended myself strongly and the result was a rift that lasted several years. Meanwhile,

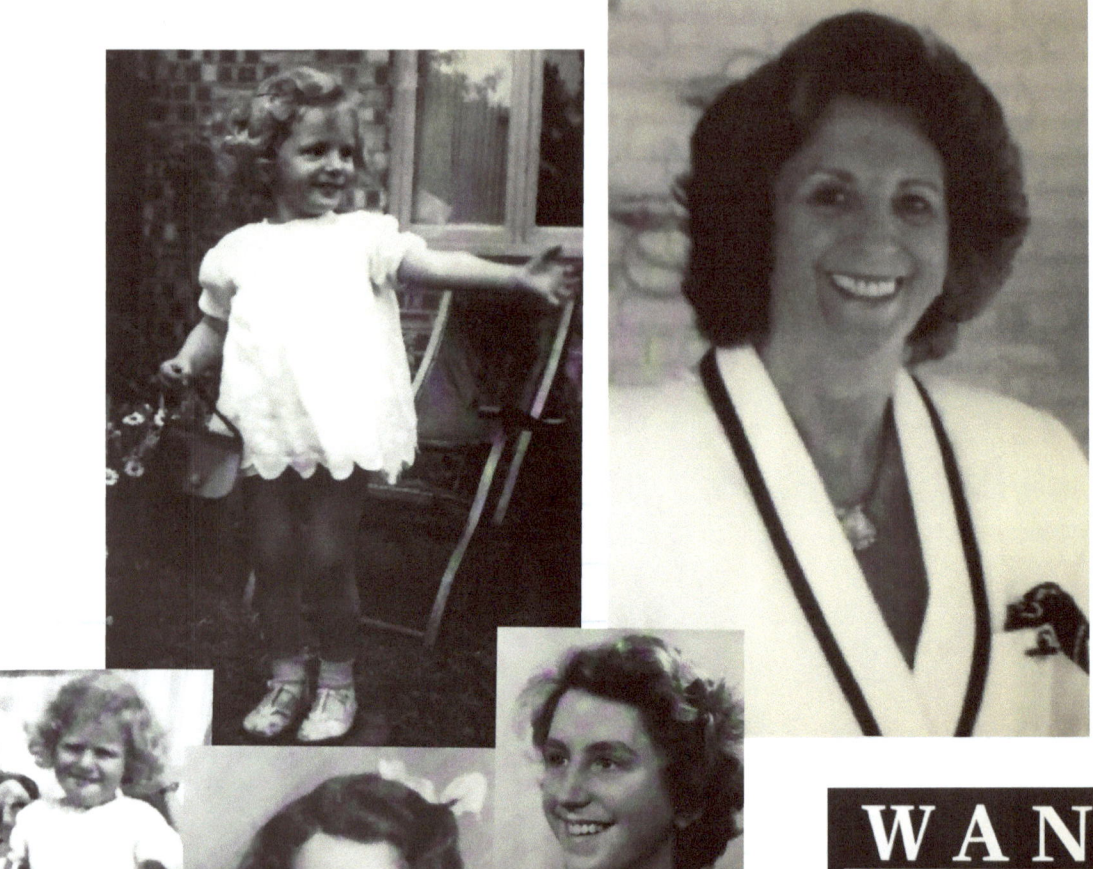

On Kathy's birthday in 1996 her friends set up a party which included having her walk down the main street where lots of stores had photos of her in the window. Here is a grouping of some of those photos. I also attach one of the most amusing, I thought, of these displays, the "Wanted" notice (right).

4

we went ahead with a neuropsychological evaluation in May, 2008. The report shocked me! Here are some excerpts:

'The patient arrived on time for her appointment. She was awake and alert. She was oriented to person, place, time and situation but she could not remember my name. When I asked her the name of the county, she gave me her zip code instead. Attention and concentration were adequate. She was well groomed and dressed. She ambulated without difficulty. No unusual motor activity. No sensory deficits. No pain behaviors. Speech was intact. Word-finding difficulties were noted. No dyspraxia. Thought processes were somewhat tangential. Content was generally appropriate. No hallucinations or delusional. Mood and affect were appropriate to the situation.'

'The patient's score of 22 on the Folstein Mini Mental Status Examination placed her on the 5th percentile for her age group. She had difficulty with both serial 7s and spelling the word 'world' backwards. Delayed recall was 0/3. On the Clox Executive Drawing Task, the patient's initial drawing was in a range typically associated with individuals who are not capable of living independently in the community.'

Rather than quoting the report word for word, here are a few interesting numbers.
- 14th percentile on the Mattis Dementia Rating Scale
- Verbal IQ 84
- Rey Auditory Verbal Learning Test below the 1st percentile
- Visual-spatial recall 17th percentile

A conclusion was that the results of the testing were consistent with a diagnosis of early Alzheimer Disease.

When she came out of the doctor's testing she was very upset. The doctor had put math questions to her and she felt this was unfair as she had never been good at math. There seemed to be little more to be said. We returned to our

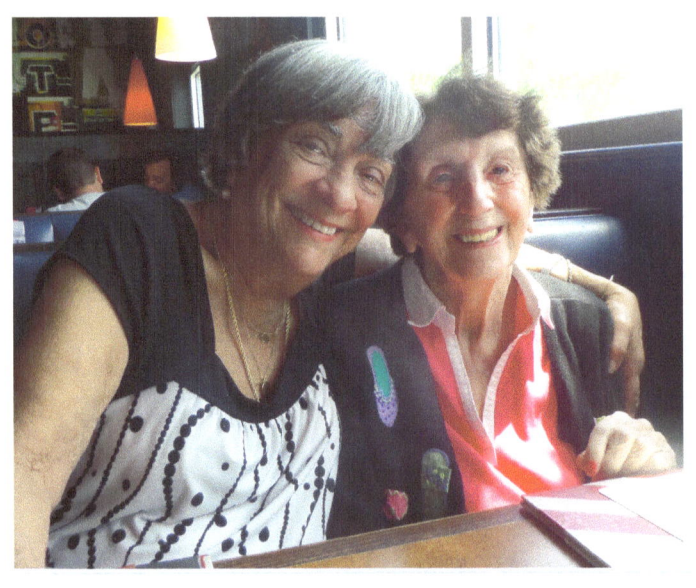

normal life and for some time nothing seemed to change much. She started several medications, though no one seemed to have much confidence in their effectiveness.

A year and a half later I started to be more aware of changes in Kathy's abilities and behavior and decided to begin keeping a record. From here onwards, I wrote notes in a sort of journal, though it was spread over nearly 6 years. Here goes:-

Jan 15, 2010

I have decided to make occasional notes on how Kathy's mental condition develops. It will just be factual observation of her memory function, her rational thinking and her use of words.

One of the oddest today was at 5.35 pm when she first read the time as 6.30 and then as 4 something. She seemed to have difficulty distinguishing the hour and minute hands.

She tries to do the crossword every day but has difficulty focusing on one clue and one answer at a time. Having done a clue she is liable to study it again 5 minutes later, forgetting that she has already done it.

April 15, 2010

At bridge last night it was her turn to open the bidding and before I could stop her she played a card instead. When we stopped her and told her we hadn't done the bidding yet, she went blank! It took us several explanations before she 'woke up' and bid.

A few weeks ago she got the supper - bacon and eggs. She called me that it was ready, so I got up to carry the plates. All there was was bacon on English muffins. No eggs. When I asked her what happened to the eggs, she went blank!

June 34, 2010

She has problems with the calendar. I am being careful to write down every possible commitment for her or me, but she keeps asking what day it is and what an entry means.

On Tuesday morning she kept on asking me when I was leaving to play golf. I kept telling her my golf was Wednesday and a few minutes later she'd ask the same question. She wouldn't accept that it was still Tuesday!

July 18, 2010

On Friday evening she came from the bedroom to the family room and said she couldn't turn the TV on. The remote wouldn't work. She showed me the remote. It was a telephone handset!

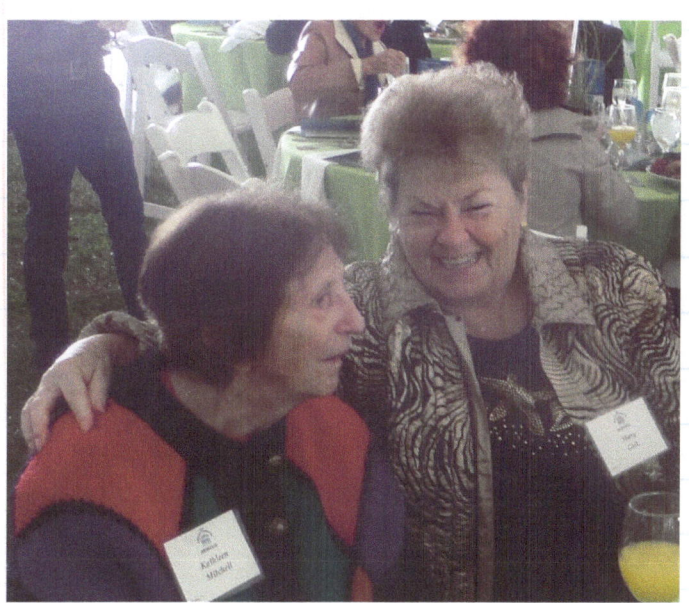

This morning she came out of the bathroom and said her blood pressure was 134.5. She asked me what that meant. I asked her when she had taken her BP and she said - just then, in the bathroom. I asked her how she had done it and she said - on that thing on the floor in the corner. I asked her if she knew what scales were for and she went blank! It took several minutes of conversation for her to remember that scales measure weight.

October 13, 2010

Her numbers problems are getting worse. Today she couldn't understand the date 10/13/10 as being October, nor recognize the final 10 as being the year.

She's becoming fixated on the calendar in an odd way! She repeatedly checks it during the day but often doesn't know what day it is and may - e.g. - think that Tuesday's events are for Monday.

The bedroom TV turns on with one red button. She usually catches another button with it, "power off", alongside the red button, but insists she didn't.

She is having problems with the piano. Her one piece is the left hand part for a duet and she's getting so that at times she can't find the first note.

{A note}

In September 2011, I was fortunate enough to be recommended to an organization called Jewish Family & Children's Service, JFCS. I learned that there were two opportunities available to me. Twice a week, on Wednesdays and Fridays, they hold meetings for caregivers. The meeting leader starts by asking an open question, "have you taken care of yourself this week?" Every participant has to answer yes or no and each one in turn reports on the good and the not-so-good of the past week. A typical meeting may be attended by 6 to 10 caregivers who give their news and, in return may get advice or sympathy from the group. I attended these meetings almost every week until March, 2013 and got unique benefit from them.

The other service was being able to call on a free caregiver for 4 hours each week. The helper who came to us hit it off beautifully with Kathy and I was able to squeeze in a weekly golf game.

The meetings stimulated me to compose the poem which appears on the back of this book and I shared it with the caregivers.

December 19, 2011

I've made no notes for a long time. In the past year she has declined steadily. She is having difficulty finding words. My deafness adds a problem - if I don't hear something and ask what she said, she usually can't remember! She is tending to hallucinate in the evenings. She will ask when "they" are leaving.

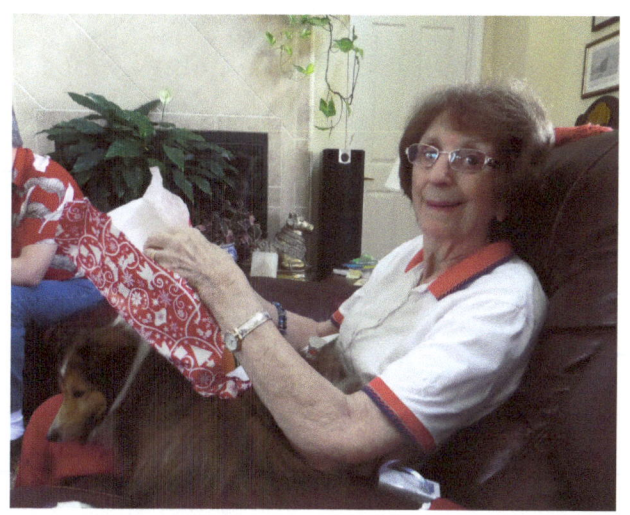

March 8, 2012

Evenings are definitely the worst. She has a tendency to put on outdoor clothes at bedtime, ready to go out, and cannot understand when I tell her it's time to put her night-clothes on.

A constant feature is an apparent need to arrange things - not all bad, but she tends to pick up and move things of mine and put them who knows where.

August 22, 2012

Today we did a lot of packing for our trip to Raleigh. Kathy turned out to be unable to put together a toiletries kit. I had to do it for her. I wish I knew more about women's toiletry kits! She has literally dozens of bottles, lipsticks etc. I found seven tooth brushes and threw out six.

October to December 2012

We joined the Annual Southbay bowling league. We were in different teams and at first Kathy was upset and wanted to be with me all the time. Her team members were very understanding and saw that they had to help her.

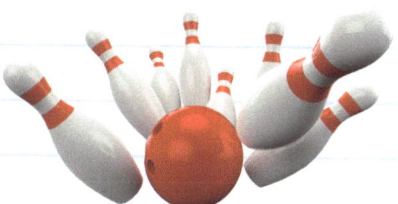

They did little things like pointing her in the right direction and she managed to get quite consistent, with the result that her team won. At the bowling banquet on December 13, they received the winners' trophy.

April 4, 2013

[In April 2013, we accepted an invitation from our son Alistair to move in with him and his wife, Jessie, rather than going on with my search for a long term care facility. The move went OK except that we were moving a full house to a

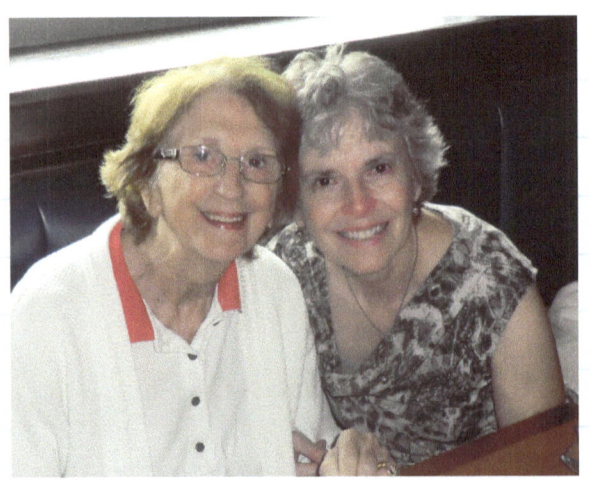

full house with the result that many of our possessions are still in boxes in the garage! But the overall result was very good and I gained an extra caregiver.]

We went together to the County office and I changed my driver's license into one with our new address. We changed Kathy's into an ID card as she had accepted that she would stop driving.

July 11, 2013

Again a long gap! One of her oddities now is taking her pants off at any time of day and wandering into the family room half naked.

Things are not helped now by the fact that we moved to Alistair's in Tampa in March and our stuff is still mostly in boxes. She did quite well on our trip to the UK in April/May.

She has a fixation on paper - folding it, throwing facial tissues in odd places ..... But she doesn't know what to do with toilet paper. I have to follow her and get rid of it after she has been to the toilet!

July 14, 2013

She is developing an odd handicap. She has difficulty recognizing an object that I point out to her.

Example: I wanted to turn off the ceiling fan and she was standing right in front of the table where the remote control was lying. When I pointed to it and asked her to bring it to me, she bent down and put her hand on some paper that was lying beside the remote. I tried for several minutes to guide her hand a few inches to the remote, but she couldn't see it or recognize it! It seems that her brain, eyes and hands are losing connection.

July 29, 2013

I more or less have to supervise both dressing and undressing. She tends to go to bed early (9:00 pm) but climbs into bed fully dressed. When I persuade her to get up, get undressed and put on her nightdress, she's liable to start putting her clothes back on if I turn my back.

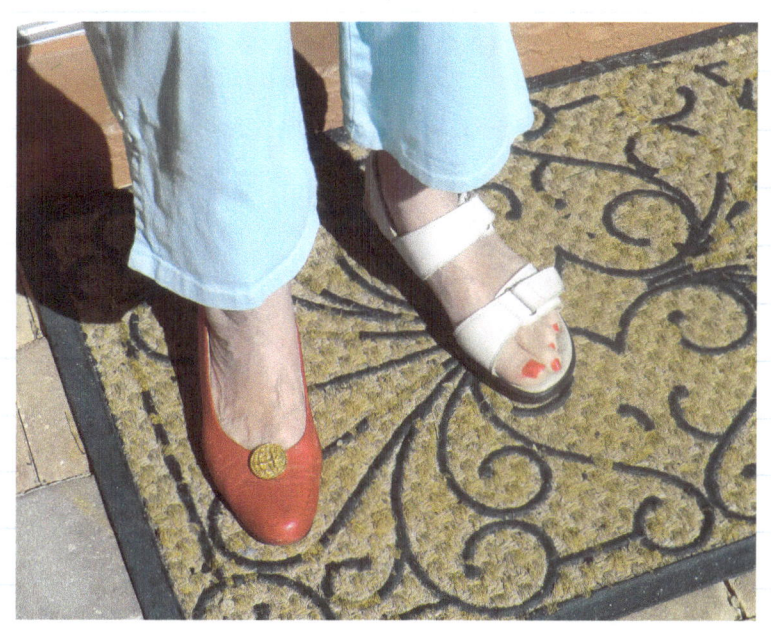

She dressed herself this morning

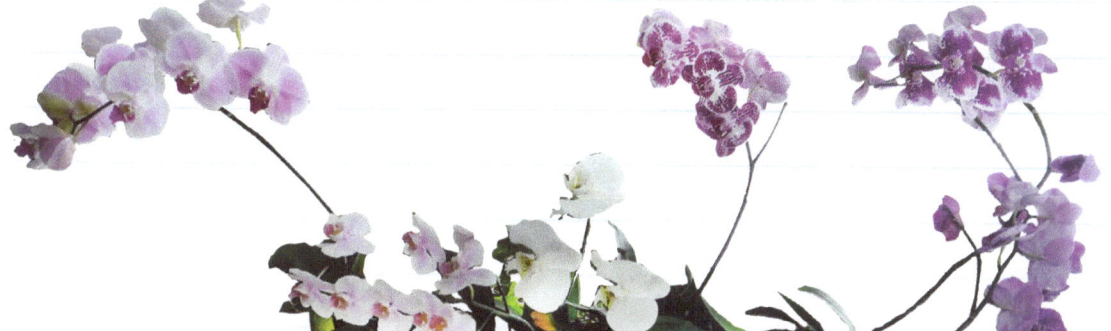

11

August 13, 2013

There is a disconnect developing between her brain and her senses - at least that's the only way I can describe it. e.g. Suppose I ask her to pass me the TV remote control, which is right in front of her. She will reach out for anything nearby - paper, a glass... I might say "move your hand to the left". She might move her hand to another object and another.... She may know, if asked, what a TV remote is, but her brain and her eyes won't link.

Now I see I tried to describe this a month ago!

September 6, 2013

She can't help picking up any papers, such as Alistair's mail or business items and then shuffling them or putting them down somewhere else. I suspect it's an urge to tidy. If I ask her or tell her not to do it, she is often upset and cries. Quite a dilemma.

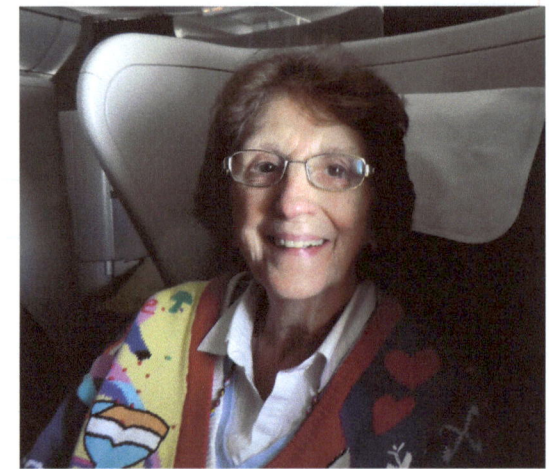

September 29, 2013

She never used to cry, but she is becoming liable to cry for almost no reason. I suspect some sort of fear.... Fear of her own inability to communicate....fear of losing me?

This morning she got up long before me and when I woke up she was fully dressed but had put her nightdress on over her clothes!

October 28, 2013

The mind/ eye/ hand disconnect is getting worse. She knows what a mug of tea looks like but it's impossible to guide her to it with words. When I point to it she looks in another direction. When I get her looking in the right direction, I can steer her hand to within an inch of the mug and she still can't pick it up.

One of the problems that affects all of us is a habit of getting up and shuffling to a position where she is exactly in front of the TV screen. Then it's almost impossible to persuade her to move!!!

November 11, 2013

Today she took off her trousers at about 5:30 pm and put on her nightdress over her shirt, followed by putting a cardigan over the lot!

January 5, 2014

She had quite a chat with Pat when I handed her the phone. She did well.

I was depressed yesterday when I realized that we will never again share memories of long ago. The "do you remember when..." is gone.

This morning she began to fiddle with my calendar and other papers beside my chair and when I gently tried to stop her she suddenly burst into anger. She has done that once or twice in the last few weeks. She can't resist playing with any pile of paper, so Alistair has to avoid leaving business papers on the living room table.

Getting her dressed or undressed is always a problem. Her brain is disconnected from her senses, so if I suggest taking off a shirt, her hands will go to her trousers. If I ask her to pass me her mug, her hands will go to something else beside it.

January 22, 2014

She has an inner drive to 'tidy' everything. Last week I found the toilet full of paper and when I tried to flush it wouldn't go. After several attempts to clear it, I found she had emptied the bathroom bin into it. The bin included a toothbrush that I had thrown out and we had to get a plumber to clear it.

She can't keep her hands off paper, so we have to watch what she does with Alistair's mail and business stuff.

In the evening she regularly goes and gets into bed fully clothed. When I follow later, she gets upset when I ask her to get up, get undressed and put on her nightdress.

February 23, 2014

This morning she got up while I was still asleep and got dressed, but she put her shirt on back-to-front!

She tends to shuffle around, pausing every now and then and doing a slight bend of her knees as if she is going to collapse. She indicates a pain in her knee, but only briefly. Does she actually have much discomfort? It's hard to tell because most of the time there is no sign of pain.

March 28, 2014

I think she's losing connection in some way between her senses (sight, hearing) and her body's ability to respond. I'll ask the doctor to refer us to a neurologist. When you call to her, she sometimes doesn't know which way to look, though you may be only a few feet from her. When you point to, e.g., an empty mug and ask her to take it to the kitchen, she may look straight at it, but moves her hand to something else, inches away from it. Her eyes don't see what you are naming.

The toilet is becoming a potential problem though she's not yet incontinent. She can wipe herself, but may bring the paper into the living room.

May 22, 2014

No major change from my last note. She seems to be crying more. Typically at about 10:00 am she will suddenly start to cry. Of course she has no idea why, or, if she does, she can't put it in words.

We normally eat supper in front of the TV with the plates on our laps. She can't hold a plate flat - always holds it tilted towards her, so she spills a lot on her shirt.

I've found that when she gets upset, if we sing "Happy Birthday" she quickly joins in and cheers up.

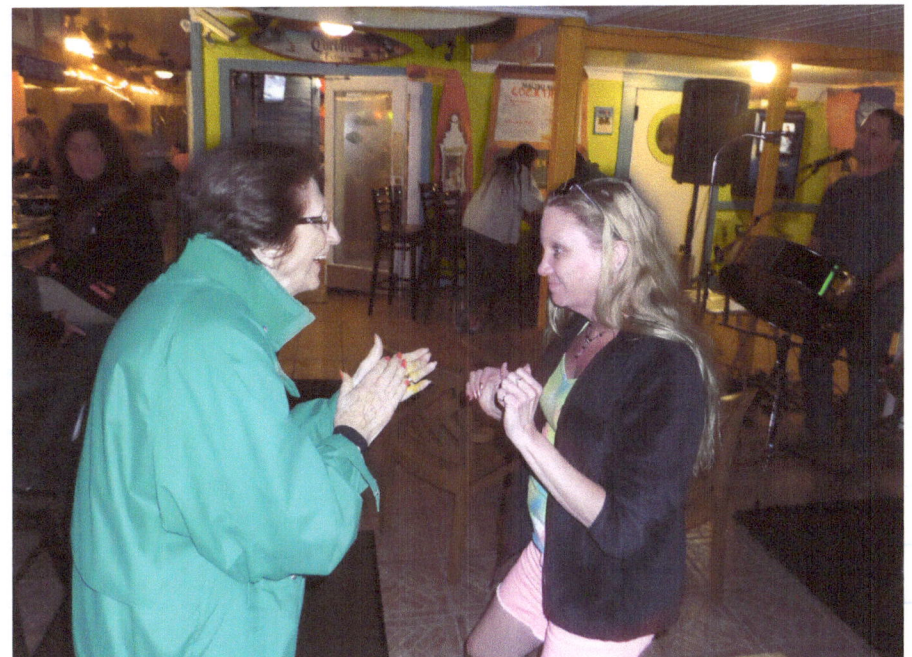

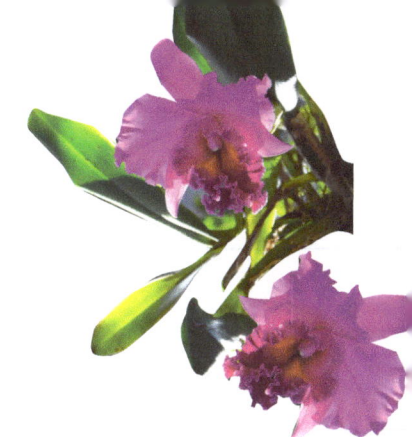

She reacts well to music. She likes to go into dance steps and gestures when Bradley plays the piano.

June 23, 2014

It seems that the part of her brain that controls motor nerves is progressively being affected. If she needs to turn in a standing position, her feet can get tangled so that she staggers. Putting on trousers can be a problem because she can't control how much to lift each leg.

She can't stay sitting down! She'll sit for one minute, get up and shuffle around, sit down again, get up again, etc. etc. The only thing that may keep her sitting for a while is playing with paper.

Lying flat gets her very agitated. She has to have her head raised by at least two pillows. At the hairdressers she got very upset when we tried to get her to lie with her head back for rinsing. Then the same thing happened at the dentist's. She couldn't let the hygienist lie her back for tooth cleaning. She gets terrified, literally!

July 14, 2014

I'm getting concerned about her taking of pills. She has 4 in the morning and 6 in the evening. I have her hold out her hand, I put the pills in it, she takes them in her mouth and I hand her a mug of water to swallow them with.

The odd question is that she has a problem with holding out her hand. I often have to take hold of it and put it flat to receive the pills. So far she's OK with then putting them in her mouth, but what would I do if she just stood there holding them? I need advice on how to get her to take her pills when she stops understanding what I'm getting her to do!

August 4, 2014

Not much change. Her inability to recognize something I point out to her is getting more pronounced. I can't ask her to pass me her glass because she doesn't see the glass. She'll pick up anything else nearby, particularly if it's paper!!

I still can't get her to lie flat in bed. She has to have her shoulders on the pillow and her head further up or else she goes into a funk.

At Jessie' suggestion, I fixed her up with my IPod and ear buds and turned on the ABBA songs. Her face lit up and she hummed along with the music and did a shuffling dance. Must do this more.

August 13, 2014

This morning when she got out of bed, she staggered around having balance problems. I had to hold her up until she got herself together. I have noticed a bit of this before - when you ask her to turn and face a different direction, she sometimes staggers in the process of turning.

She is beginning to have slight incontinence. A couple of nights ago she got up during the night to go for a pee and I later found a small pool of what I think was pee on the bathroom floor. I have started putting pads in her underwear.

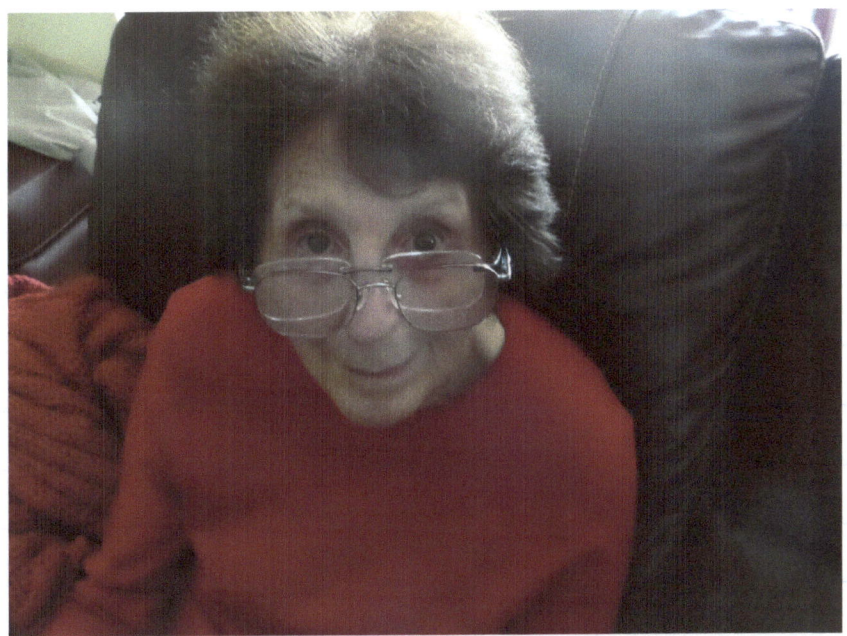
So that's where my glasses went

September 1, 2014

An odd little quirk that I have just noticed, but I think it has been developing. When she wants to move to one side, say left, she moves the right foot first, bumps it into the left foot, stumbles and nearly falls over. I've had to catch her several times. I had thought it was a balance problem but now I think it's a coordination problem.

October 12, 2014

I don't think she has much reasoning power left. When I help her in the toilet, if she wipes herself (I do it for her often) I try to remind her to drop the paper in the bowl. She always now brings it out and drops it on the floor.

Her fixation on paper is increasing. She pulls dozens of tissues from the box and then tears them into small pieces which mostly end up on the carpet.

She still likes magazines, but can't read them. I find them with tissues stuffed between the pages.

We nearly had a nasty accident due to her lack of understanding. After I had loaded our grocery shopping into the Buick, I went to shut the tailgate. Luckily I saw she had her hand on the pillar where the tailgate would have crushed it, so I told her to move her hand. She didn't move so I had to grab her hand and move it for her.

December 4, 2014

Not much measurable change. Getting her dressed can be difficult because she doesn't understand "lift up your leg".

Getting her to lay her head on the pillow at bed-time can also be oddly difficult. It's the same as when she has to put her head back into a washbasin at the hairdressers to have the dye rinsed. She seems to fear having her head back. I see I recorded this in June.

We had a visit by Julian and family over Thanksgiving and she did quite well - I think! I don't actually think she recognized anyone!

December 21, 2014

I think she does have a balance problem, though she's better at standing on one leg than I am.

Eating is another problem. She can't hold a plate flat so her food is always on the verge of pouring into her lap. She also tends to get up when she has eaten half, for no apparent reason. She eats the rest quite happily as long as I feed it to her.

She has more and more difficulty walking. She shuffles in a bent-over posture and if we go any distance she starts to get collapsing knees. She doesn't fall. You just have to take a pause.

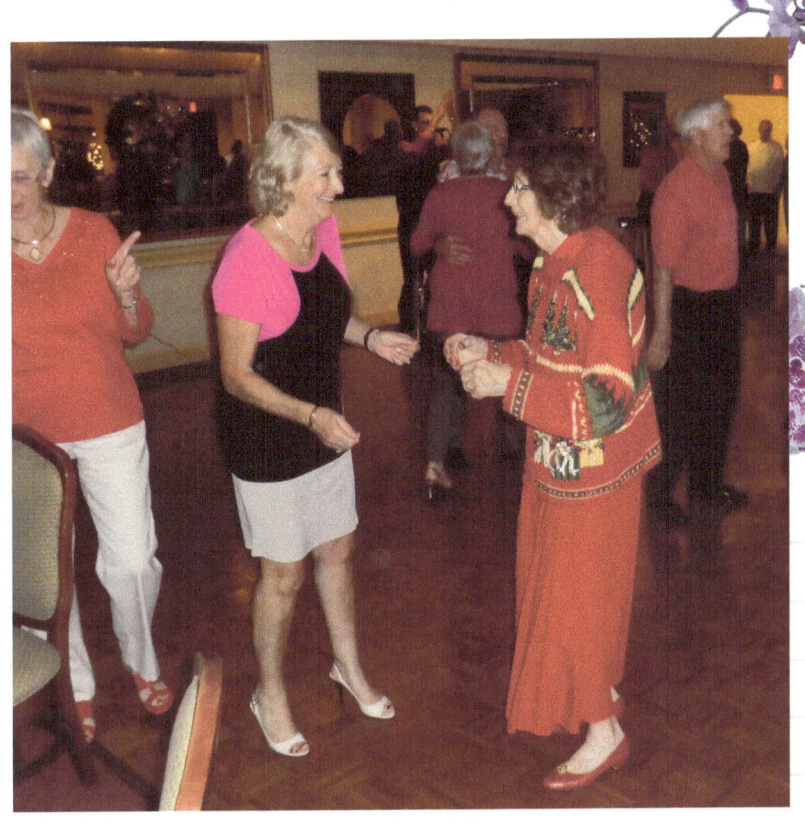

Music gets her dancing

February 9, 2015

Not much new to report. The balance problem is growing and she's liable to fall over if she touches her toe against anything.

Her incontinence is increasing. Her Depend panties usually get urine in them between visits to the toilet. If she goes for a pee on her own, she doesn't get her back properly lined up and has peed on the rug more than once.

It's also getting harder to communicate with her. If I tell her it's bed-time when she's facing away from me, it's hard to get her to turn around. She'll walk the way she's facing!

February 18, 2015

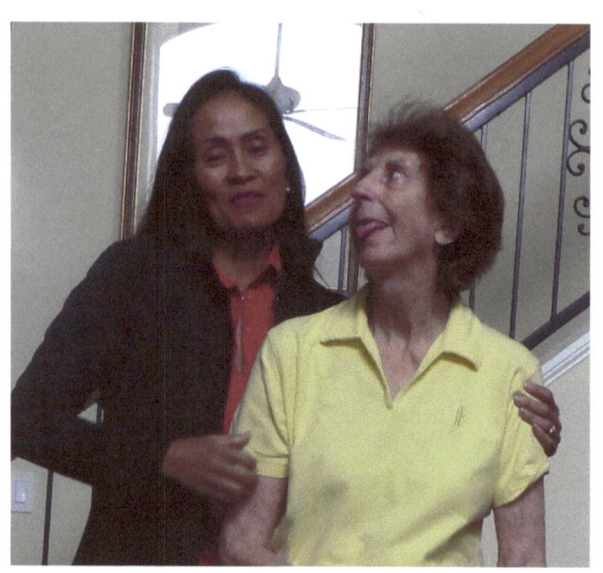

Yesterday she fell by the sofa and nearly did the same again today. It's because, when she wants to sit down, she doesn't point her back at the seat. She turns half way and then sits half-on, half-off. I've spotted this in time several times and avoided her ending on the floor. At least she doesn't hurt herself with this maneuver because she doesn't have far to go as she slides off.

February 21, 2015

Her balance and walking are definitely getting shakier. She fell again a couple of days ago because she turned only half way to sit on the sofa and missed.

Also her incontinence is increasing. I now fit her day and night with diapers but she still managed to wet the bed 4 days ago - she had filled and over flowed the diaper during the night.

March 10, 2015

I don't think I have fully mentioned before how she can no longer dress herself. I always offer her her trousers to put on by herself, but she tends to put a foot in the wrong leg, or not get it into a leg at all! I have to put on her sweaters or shirts, though she's not bad at doing up buttons.

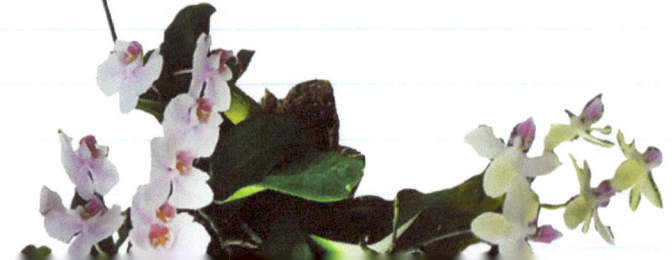

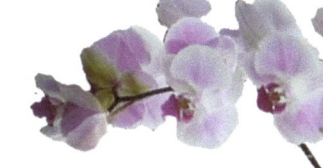

March 23, 2015

She has developed a compulsion which makes getting her dressed and undressed quite difficult. Her fingers grab hold of things she touches - such as sleeves or panties. Helping her take off a shirt comes to a halt when she won't take her arm out of a sleeve. When I try to make her let go, she gets cross and swings at me. She never actually hits me, it's just a gesture.

April 6, 2015

Her hearing has an odd quirk. If I call her she seems unable to track where my voice came from. I have to call several times before she will turn toward me.

She cries a lot these days for no apparent reason. She also sleeps a lot on the sofa or back in bed at any time of day.

May 3, 2015

The night before last at 4:00 am she fell out of bed with a loud crash. It took me some moments to disentangle myself from the sheets, but I finally got round to where she was lying in a heap on the floor. It cost me quite an effort to get her up, and I decided to help her to the toilet in case that was what started things.

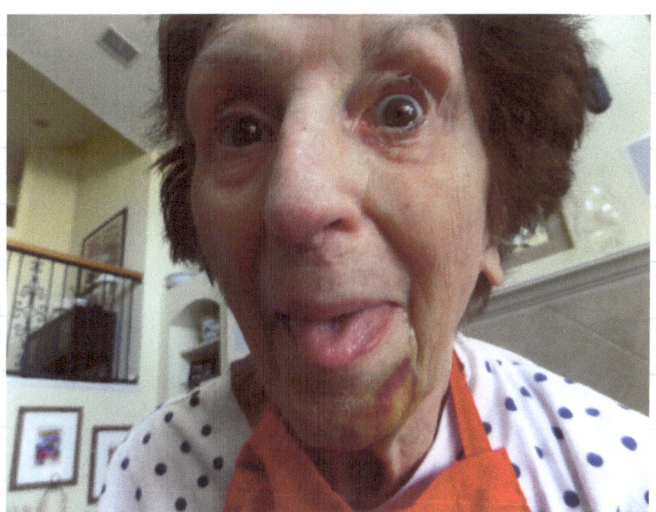

She obviously banged her chin against the night stand beside the bed and she has a vivid bruise on her chin. It looks like the result of one of my right hooks!

May 21, 2015

She is getting worse at feeding herself. I always try to leave her to it and she manages if it's something that can involve a spoon, but even then she tends to drop food in her lap. If it's the kind of pasta that needs a fork, she has difficulty pushing the fork in. She eats her morning cereal but makes a bit of a mess.

Her balance is now very poor. She shuffles around in a deep hunch and we have to watch in case she catches her foot against something and nearly falls.

She has an interesting bias to the left. When she sits down she always slumps to the left and dozes off. When I am walking her to bed or the toilet, I always have to keep turning her away from the left.

May 24, 2015

The finger grab that I described on March 23 is very strong. Anything she touches her fingers hook on and don't let go. If I need her to let go, as in undressing her for bed, I have to rip the garment away by force, because she doesn't understand a request. If I do rip she doesn't get upset.

I have evolved a routine to get her into bed without her resisting putting her head down. I pull the sheet and blanket well down the bed and sit her on the bed, about half way down. I help her get as far up on the bed as possible and then lower her sideways onto the pillow. This avoids the problem of putting the back of her head down, see the funk reported on June 23, 2014. Once she is comfortable, I sing her the lullaby "Golden slumbers..." And she seems to go to sleep while I sing!

July 1, 2015

I've just looked back over several years of notes and see that I have covered just about every aspect of her deterioration. Now it's more or less the same things just getting worse. Probably the most difficult problem now is her incontinence.

I think she has lost all bladder and rectal control, so we have to take her to the toilet at short intervals and change her diapers more frequently.

July 10, 1015

I have to be thankful for small bright spots. Recently when I tucked her into bed and said "I love you" she said it back to me in a firm, clear voice. This morning she ate her cereal without spilling any.

I see that it's only a year or so since she started being incontinent. It's manageable but it's putting a strain on my back, having to lower her on the bowl, lift her off and bend to lift up her diapers and trousers - and my knees are complaining!

August 14, 2015

I have noted her balance problem before but it is getting really bad. When I get her up from bed or sitting, I have to hold her up for a while until she more or less stabilizes herself. 3 days ago she fell, apparently when trying to sit on a little stool in the bathroom. It was 5:00 am and I was woken by a huge crash. She had a cut on her left temple, perhaps hitting against the bathroom door. It took me a lot of strength to get her up. I washed the cut and found a band-aid for it. The stool was on its side.

September 7, 2015

Yesterday I heard an odd sound from the bedroom and found she had fallen. I got her up and couldn't find any cuts or bruises, but when I tried to take her to the bathroom, she was really limping - holding no weight on her right leg. She woke me at 3:30 am and I had another tough time taking her to the bathroom. I don't think she went back to sleep at all and I had the same battle again in the morning.

I reported the whole tale to Jessie and she helped me from then on. We used the wheel chair from then. The problem seems to be her hip. We have a doctor's appointment tomorrow and I'll see if we can get her an X-ray.

September 8, 2015 and subsequent days

Turned out she had fractured her right hip. We went from the doctor's office to our nearest hospital, Tampa Community Hospital. They repaired her hip surgically on the 9th.

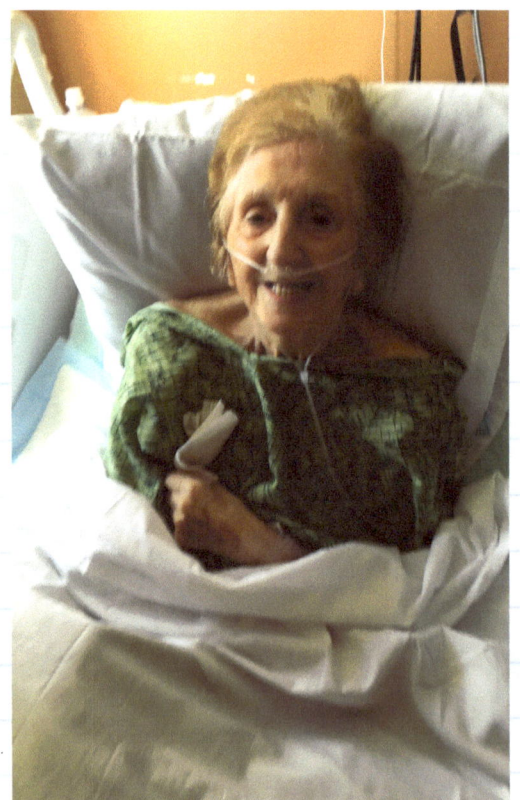 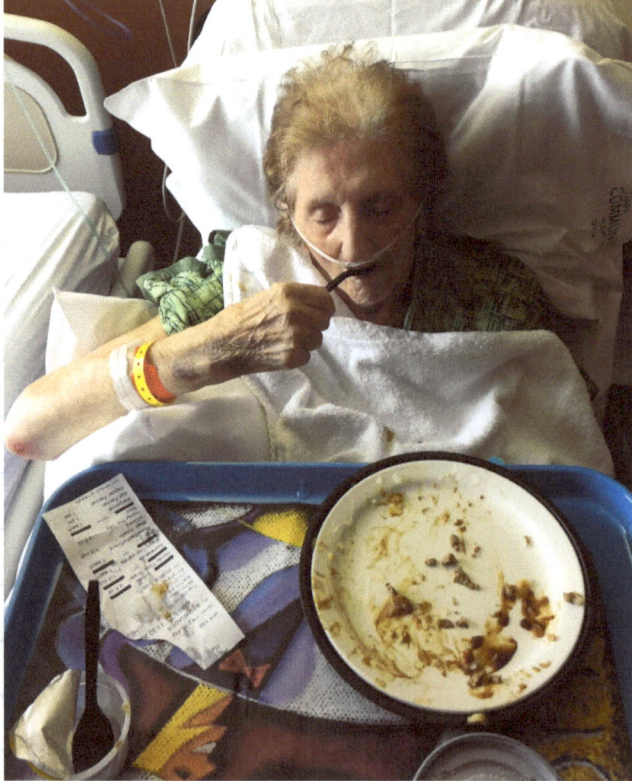

Recovering at the hospital in September

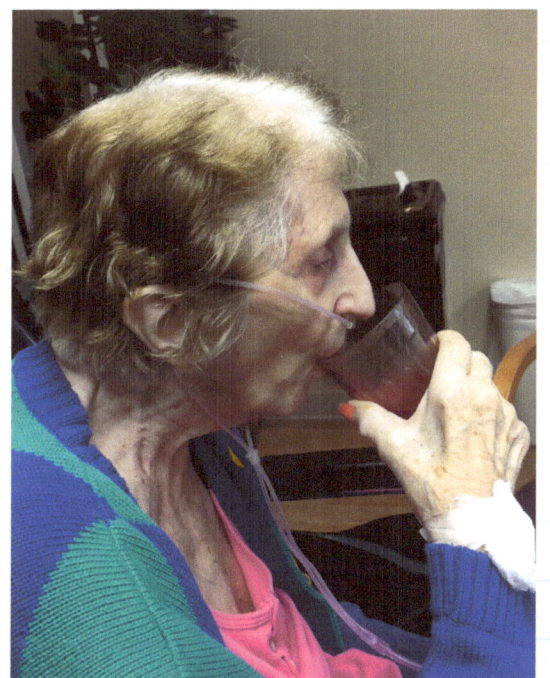
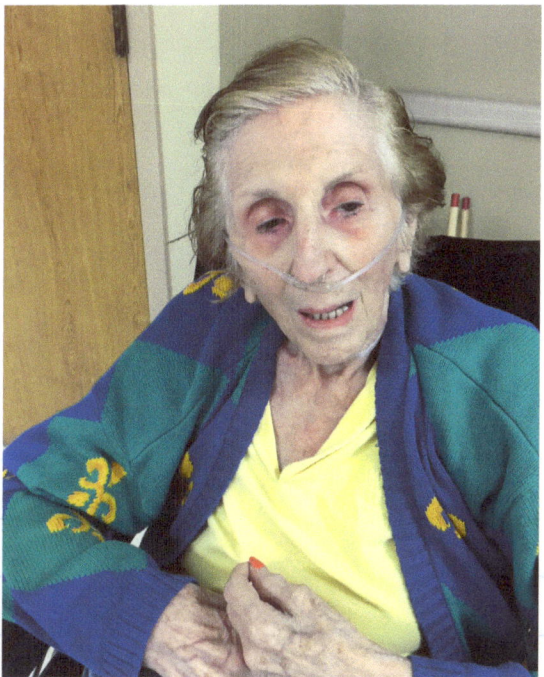
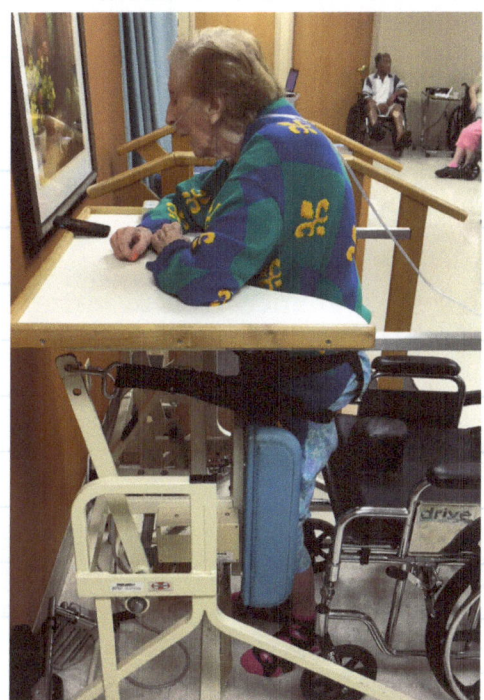
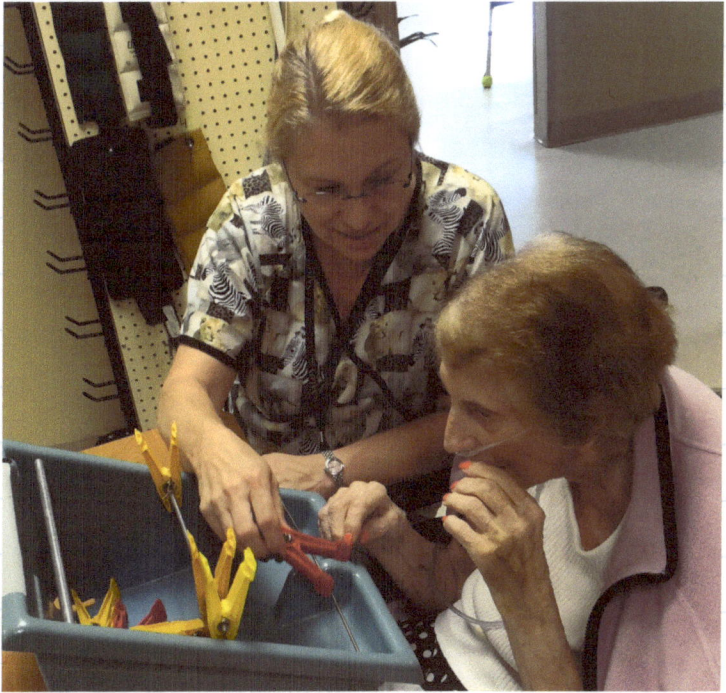

The rehab techs did their best to get Kathy to work, but she did not respond.

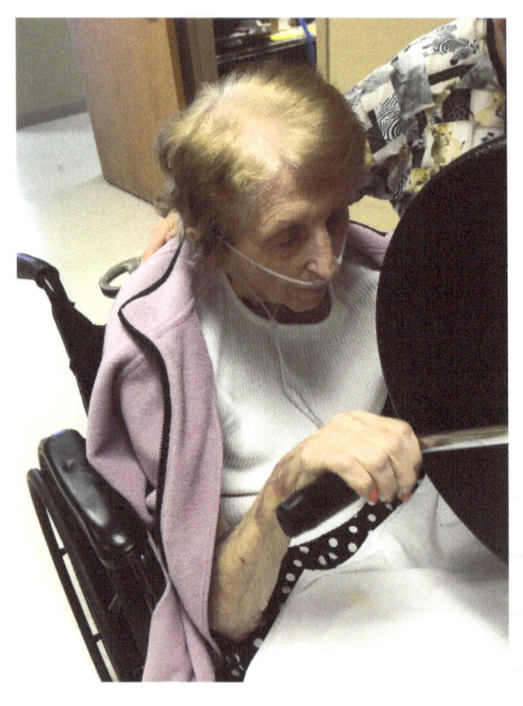

After surgery

She then spent five days in the hospital during which she got partially back to where she was before - eating and drinking but no physical activity.

September 15, 2015

We moved her to Brandon Health and Rehabilitation Center. She continued to do okay for a while, though when they tried to get her active on several exercises, she reacted passively. She was unable to understand instructions and remained immobile at whatever machine or game they had put her in.

She developed a urinary tract infection with a high fever and was taken to Brandon Hospital. She returned to rehab but went steadily downhill. On the 30th she was found to have an excess sodium level and went back to the hospital. By this time she had more or less stopped eating and drinking and we were faced with the decision not to take forced action. Kathy and I had reached that agreement years ago, so on October 7th we had her brought home in Hospice care and she died quietly on October 10th.

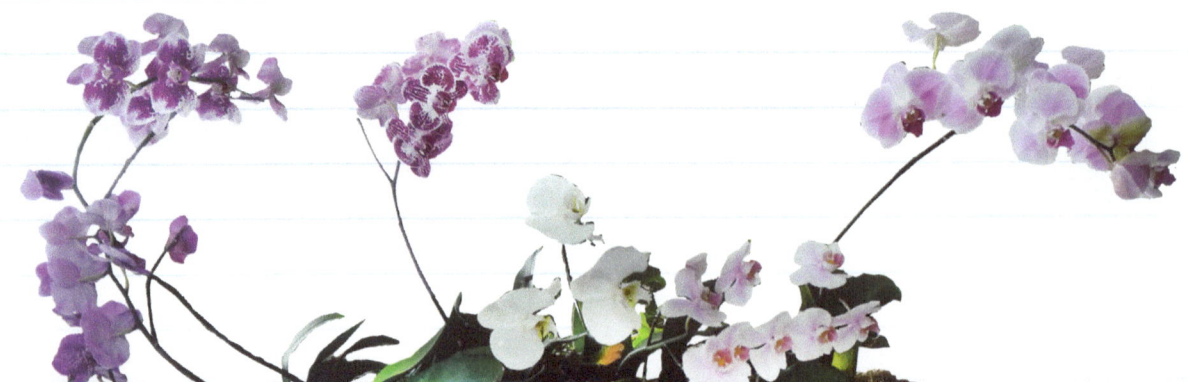

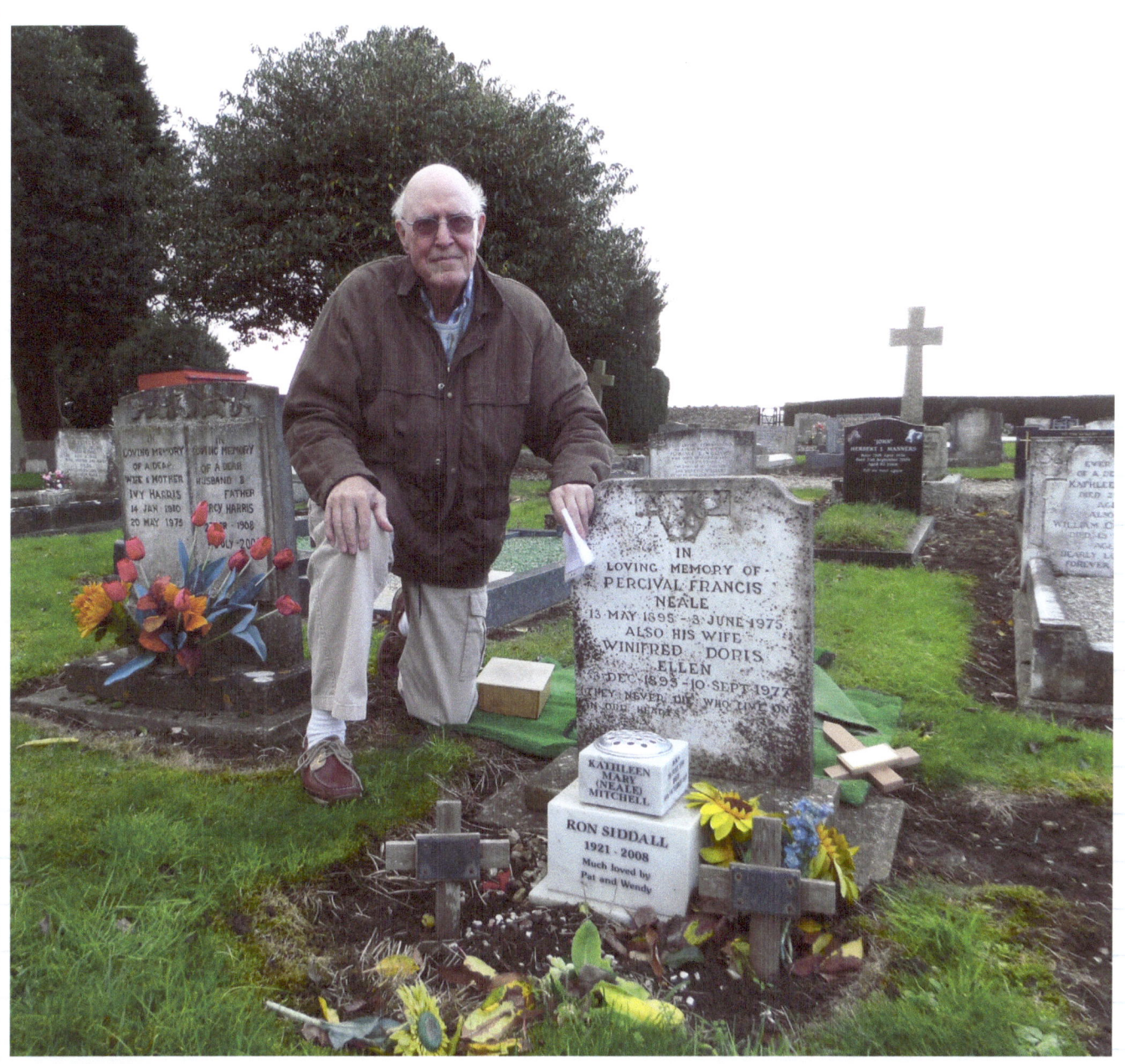

I laid her to rest with her parents in England